I0838820

Diabetes Cookbook For Newly Diagnosed Men

The Complete Guide to Managing Diabetes In Men

Mclan O. Micheals, RDN

Disclaimer

The information provided in this guide is for educational purposes only and should not replace professional medical advice. Always consult with your healthcare provider for personalized guidance and recommendations related to your specific circumstances.

     Mclan O. Micheals, RDN.

Copyright © 2023, Mclan O. Micheals, RDN

All rights reserved.

No part of this book may be reproduced or transmitted in any form or by any means, electronic or mechanical, including photocopying, recording, or any information storage or retrieval system, without written permission from the author.

Table of Contents

Introduction

We set out on a culinary adventure that involves more than simply treating diabetes; it's about enjoying a full life, one that includes wonderful meals and a rekindled feeling of well-being.

Think about Mark, who is in his mid-40s and has a full schedule with his job, family, and other obligations. Mark receives the news that changes everything one day: he has been given a diabetes diagnosis. His environment is now full of doubt, issues, and the need to drastically alter his way of life.

Like many people who have just received a diagnosis, Mark was confused and overwhelmed by the challenges of managing his diabetes. But instead of giving in to hopelessness, he made the decision to consider it a chance for development, a chance to take control of his health, and an invitation to investigate the power of nutrition.

The insight that controlling diabetes is not about deprivation or sacrifice, but rather about making

      Mclan O. Micheals, RDN.

educated decisions, finding balance, and appreciating every meal along the way, was the beginning of Mark's journey, just like yours. He learned that he could use food as a tool to manage his blood sugar, fuel his body, and satiate his spirit.

This cookbook was created as a result of Mark's experience, a monument to the power of food to improve the lives of newly diagnosed diabetic males. It is a carefully chosen collection of recipes, ideas, and advice that addresses the particular requirements and issues that men with diabetes could face.

You will discover a wealth of delectable, diabetes-friendly recipes that will suit a variety of tastes and preferences inside these pages. We have you covered for everything from filling breakfasts to healthy lunches, robust dinners, and even decadent desserts. Each recipe has been painstakingly created to establish the ideal balance between flavor and nutrition, guaranteeing that flavor is never sacrificed.

You will learn useful techniques for meal planning and eating out, as well as information

        Mclan O. Micheals, RDN.

on portion management, reading labels, and understanding carbs. To live a full and active life while managing your diabetes, we want you to feel empowered to make wise dietary choices.

Please keep in mind that this cookbook is not intended to replace professional medical advice or tailored treatment from your healthcare team. It is intended to supplement their knowledge and act as a resource to enable you to get the most out of your path toward managing your diabetes. Together with your healthcare providers, you may develop a personalized plan that addresses your particular requirements and promotes your long-term well-being.

This book is for anybody who wants to adopt a healthy lifestyle, whether they are a newly diagnosed man searching for assistance, a caregiver looking for nourishing meals for a loved one, or someone who is enthusiastic about doing so. Let's go on a culinary journey together that honors the ability of food to nourish, heal, and transform lives.

Let the "Diabetes Cookbook for Newly Diagnosed Men" be your dependable travel partner as you embark on this amazing quest for a delectable and healthy lifestyle. One delicious dish at a time, embrace the tastes, appreciate the moments, and take charge of your health. The rewards are incalculable, and the possibilities are limitless.

Ready to join us now? Turn the page, and let's explore the world of cooking for people with diabetes together.

Chapter One

Understanding Diabetes

You've come to the correct spot if you've just received a diagnosis, have been battling type 1 or type 2 diabetes for some time, or are supporting a loved one. With all the tools, health advice, and meal suggestions you need, this is the beginning of developing a better knowledge of how you may lead a healthy life. Whatever stage your diabetes is at, remember that you have choices and that you don't have to be restricted.

Type 1

What you should know about type 1 diabetes is provided below. Every age, every ethnicity, and every shape and size is susceptible to type 1 diabetes. Having it is not shameful, and you have a network of individuals who are willing to assist you. Working together with your diabetes care team and learning as much as you can about it can provide you with all you need to flourish.

Your body converts the carbs you consume into blood glucose (also known as blood sugar), which it utilizes as fuel. Everyone can learn to control their disease and live long, healthy lives with the use of insulin therapy and other therapies.

Keep in mind that this illness is treatable. You may live a regular life and accomplish what you set out to achieve by leading a healthy lifestyle that includes exercise and a balanced diet.

Type 2

The most prevalent kind of diabetes, type 2, is characterized by improper insulin utilization by the body. While some individuals can maintain their blood glucose levels with a balanced diet and regular exercise, others may need medication or insulin to do so. In any case, you have alternatives, and we're here to provide the information, tools, and assistance you need.

Keeping a healthy diet consistent is essential for treating type 2 diabetes. You need to consume something nutritious that will improve your health while also satisfying your hunger. Recall that it is a process. Find the diet strategies and helpful hints that best fit your way of life and how to make the most of your dietary intake.

A further element of controlling type 2 is fitness. The good news is that all you need to do is start moving. The secret is to engage in things you like as often as you can. No matter how physically strong you are, a little exercise each day may help you take control of your life.

Gestational Diabetes

Although a diagnosis of gestational diabetes might be frightening, you can still control it. It doesn't always follow that you had diabetes before becoming pregnant or that you will continue to have it after giving birth. It implies that you may have a healthy pregnancy and a healthy baby by working with your doctor. Know that you have all the support you need to be at your best for both you and your baby, no matter what.

Although we are unsure of the exact etiology of gestational diabetes, we do know you are not alone. Millions of women experience it. We are aware that the placenta sustains the developing fetus. In certain cases, these hormones also prevent the mother's insulin from working properly in her body, leading to a condition known as insulin resistance. The mother's body

     Mclan O. Micheals, RDN.

finds it challenging to use insulin as a result of her insulin resistance. She may thus need up to three times as much insulin to make up for this.

Even though gestational diabetes is manageable, it may still harm you and your unborn child, so it's important to take action right away. Work with your doctor to maintain normal blood glucose levels with specialized meal programs and frequent exercise. Insulin injections and routine blood glucose tests may also be part of your therapy.

Importance of Diet in Diabetes Management

Depending on how it affects the body's capacity to metabolize glucose, food may either encourage diabetes or help avoid it.

People should stay away from processed foods, foods heavy in saturated or trans fats, foods with added sugars and syrups, and foods that elevate cholesterol and produce a sharp rise in blood sugar levels.

Processed meals and foods heavy in fat or sugar may cause inflammation by upsetting the normal relationship between glucose and insulin, but they can also increase risk factors like being overweight. It's crucial to be aware of things to avoid if you have diabetes.

Carbs must also be monitored. While all carbs are required for the body to function, some elevate blood glucose levels more than others.

Foods with a low glycemic index boost blood sugar levels gradually while sustaining satiety. On the other side, high GI meals include those that suddenly increase blood sugar levels and don't sufficiently fill the stomach.

There is no particular diet for diabetes. The key is to stick to a meal plan that suits your tastes and lifestyle and aids in achieving your blood sugar, cholesterol, triglyceride, blood pressure, and weight management objectives.

A healthy diet for anyone might be considered a diabetes diet. Eat small, frequent meals to prevent gaining weight, and be sure to

eat broccoli, mushrooms, green vegetables, apples, oranges, pear, watermelon, pineapple, guavas, and other fruits and vegetables with a low glycemic index. Be rigorous with mangoes, grapes, chikoos, and bananas. Fish, lean meat cuts, beans and lentils, and liquid oils are all better choices than processed carbohydrates.

Limit your intake of trans fats, as well as high-calorie snacks and sweets like chips, cake, and ice cream.

Diabetics Diet Rules

Planning a diabetes diet involves more than just "what one eats," It also involves timing.

There shouldn't be a lot of time between meals. The body's glucose levels might become unstable after a delay of more than three hours, which is risky for diabetics.
One may keep an eye on the levels and their effects by routinely checking their blood sugar levels before bed and after waking up.

It is advised to consume some long-acting carbohydrates before going to bed if one checks their blood sugar at night and discovers that it is low, for instance, below 6 millimoles. This will help avoid nighttime hypoglycemia.

Therefore, it is important to monitor not only the number or quality of meals but also the times at which they are consumed.

A diabetic may enjoy a normal life and keep their diabetes under control with the aid of a well-planned diabetes diet and appropriate adherence to these rules!

Cooking for Diabetes: Tips and Guidelines

A balanced diet is essential for managing diabetes properly as well as for maintaining a healthy weight, regulating blood pressure, and avoiding heart disease and stroke.

To gain tips on creating and preparing nutritious meals, always see a trained dietitian or member of your healthcare team.

To reduce calorie consumption, fat intake, and sugar intake, try these healthy cooking tips:

Instead of using butter, shortening, or oil, use nonstick cooking spray.

Choose olive, avocado, maize, peanut, sunflower, safflower, vegetable, or flaxseed oil if you do use oil.

Instead of salt, butter, or sweet sauces, season meals like meats and steamed vegetables with herbs and spices (including pepper, cinnamon, and oregano), vinegar, lemon juice, or salsa.

     Mclan O. Micheals, RDN.

On toast, use jam with reduced or no sugar instead of butter or margarine.

You should consume more omega-3 fatty acids. Get at least two servings of omega-3-rich meals each week. These include albacore tuna, salmon, sardines, mackerel, herring, and rainbow trout. Other omega-3-rich foods that may be included in a balanced diet include walnuts, flaxseed, and soy products.

Consume oatmeal or whole-grain cereals rich in fiber together with skim or 1% milk.

Replace full-fat versions of dairy products, including milk, yogurt, cottage cheese, and sour cream, with low-fat or fat-free alternatives.

Ingest pure fruit juice without any sugar added. And keep your serving sizes small.

Eat chicken or turkey without the skin and trim off any extra fat from the flesh.

Always use lean meat cuts, and prepare your food healthfully by broiling, roasting, stir-frying, or grilling.

Instead of cereals and loaves of bread prepared with refined, processed grains like white flour, choose whole-grain versions.

Healthcare experts may point you in the direction of useful websites that go into greater detail about meal planning, provide healthy recipes and cooking instructions, recommend exercise regimens, provide advice on how to control your weight, and more.

Chapter Two

Breakfast Recipes

A Balanced Breakfast Bowl

Ingredients:

Greek yogurt, one cup

Oats, rolled, in a cup

Chia seeds, one tablespoon

Fresh berries, such as strawberries, blueberries, or raspberries, to the tune of 1/4 cup

1 tablespoon of maple syrup or honey

1 tablespoon of nuts or seeds, such as pumpkin seeds, almonds, or walnuts

1 tablespoon of optionally added coconut shreds

A dash of cinnamon, if desired

Method:

- Greek yogurt, rolled oats, and chia seeds should all be combined in a dish.

- The chia seeds need time to absorb the liquid, so mix well and set it aside for 5 minutes.
- Fresh berries, honey or maple syrup, and chopped nuts or seeds should be added on top of the mixture.
- Shredded coconut and a dash of cinnamon may be added for taste if preferred.
- Combine everything, then enjoy your nutritious breakfast bowl!

Vegetable Omelette

Ingredients:

2 eggs

Any color diced bell peppers, 1/4 cup

Onions, diced, 1/4 cup

Tomato dice, one-fourth cup

1/4 cup of chopped kale or spinach

Pepper and salt as desired

1 tablespoon butter or olive oil

     Mclan O. Micheals, RDN.

Method:

- In a bowl, beat the eggs well. Add salt and pepper to taste.
- In a non-stick pan, heat butter or olive oil over medium heat.
- To the pan, add the diced bell peppers, onions, and tomatoes. Sauté for 2 to 3 minutes, or until softened somewhat.
- To the pan, add the chopped spinach or kale, and heat for an additional minute, or until wilted.
- Over the veggies in the pan, pour the beaten eggs.
- Once the bottom settles, let the eggs boil undisturbed for a few minutes.
- To enable the raw eggs to flow to the edges, gently raise the omelet's edges with a spatula and tilt the pan.
- When the omelette is about done, use a spatula to delicately turn it over, or fold it in half.

- The eggs must cook for one more minute to completely set.
- Serve the hot veggie omelet by sliding it onto a platter.

Whole-grain Pancakes

Ingredients:

whole wheat flour, 1 cup

1 teaspoon of sugar

One tablespoon of baking powder

A half-teaspoon of baking soda

1 cup buttermilk (or other milk of your choice)

and 1/4 teaspoon salt

1 egg

1 tablespoon of melted oil or butter

Optional: One-half teaspoon of vanilla extract

Method:

- Mix the whole wheat flour, sugar, baking soda, baking powder, and salt in a big bowl.

- Buttermilk, eggs, melted butter or oil, and vanilla extract (if used) should all be combined in a separate basin.

- After adding the liquid components, mix the dry ingredients just until they are barely blended.

- To let the whole wheat flour absorb the liquid, let the batter sit for 5 to 10 minutes.

- Grease a nonstick pan or griddle with butter or oil before heating it up on medium heat.

- 1/4 cup of batter should be added to the pan for each pancake. Cook the first side until surface bubbles emerge, then flip it over and cook the second side until brown.

- Continue by using the remaining batter.

- Warm whole-grain pancakes may be served with your preferred toppings, such as yogurt, fresh fruit, or maple syrup.

Avocado Toast with Poached Eggs

Ingredients:

2 toasty pieces of whole-grain bread

1 mature avocado

2 eggs

Pepper and salt as desired

Chili flakes and chopped herbs (such as parsley or cilantro) are optional garnishes.

Method:

- Remove the pit from the avocado by cutting it in half. Using a fork, mash the flesh until it is smooth after scooping it into a bowl.
- Add salt and pepper to taste and season the mashed avocado.
- By heating a saucepan of water to a low simmer, you may poach the eggs. Each

egg should be cracked into a different little dish or ramekin.

- Use a spoon to stir the simmering water into a soft whirlpool. Slide one egg slowly into the whirlpool's center. Continue by using the second egg.
- The eggs should be poached for three to four minutes so that the whites are set but the yolks are still runny.
- Spread the mashed avocado equally onto the toasted bread pieces while the eggs are poaching.
- With the use of a slotted spoon, gently remove the cooked eggs from the water, and then top the avocado toast with them.
- Add salt, pepper, and any other toppings that you choose.
- Warm avocado toast with poached eggs should be served right away.

     Mclan O. Micheals, RDN.

Chapter Three

Lunch Recipes

Salad with Grilled Chicken

Ingredients:

2 skinless, boneless chicken breasts

Pepper and salt as desired

Mixed salad greens in 6 cups

1 cup halved cherry tomatoes

1 thinly sliced cucumber

1/4 thinly sliced red Onion

1/4 cup of almond slices

1/4 cup feta cheese crumbles

Your preferred dressing, such as a lemon herb dressing or a balsamic vinaigrette.

Method

- Place a grill pan to a high temperature.
- Chicken breasts should be salted and peppered.

- Grill the chicken for 6 to 8 minutes on each side, or until it is well done and the middle is no longer pink.
- After taking the chicken from the grill, give it some time to rest before slicing it into thin strips.
- Combine the mixed salad greens, cucumber, red onion, cherry tomatoes, sliced almonds, and crumbled feta cheese in a big bowl.
- Add the chicken strips that you cooked to the salad.
- Choose your preferred dressing and drizzle it over the salad. Gently toss to incorporate.
- The grilled chicken salad should be served right away.

Wrap with Turkey and Vegetables

Ingredients:

4 substantial tortilla wraps

8 turkey breast slices

50 ml of hummus

Baby spinach leaves, 1 cup

Cup of grated carrots

Sliced cucumbers in a cup

Pepper and salt as desired

Method

- The tortilla wraps should be spread out on a spotless surface.
- Each tortilla should have a uniform coating of hummus on it.
- Each tortilla should have 2 pieces of turkey breast on it.
- Add a few baby spinach leaves, shredded carrots, and cucumber slices on top.
- Add salt and pepper to taste.
- Starting at the bottom, fold the tortilla's sides in and wrap it up firmly.

- Serve each wrap after cutting it in half diagonally.

Lentil Soup with Spinach

Ingredients:

1 cup dry lentils, washed

1 onion; chopped

2 carrots diced

2 celery stalks diced

4 cups of veggie broth

2-cups of water

Bay leaf, one

One tablespoon of dried thyme

1 teaspoon of cumin, ground

Paprika, half a teaspoon

4 cups fresh leaves of spinach

Pepper and salt as desired

(Optional) Lemon wedges for serving

Method

- A tablespoon of oil should be heated in a large saucepan over medium heat.

- Add the diced celery, carrots, and onion, all chopped. Vegetables should be sautéed for around 5 minutes until they start to soften.

- Add the ground cumin, paprika, dried thyme, and chopped garlic. Cook the mixture for one more minute, or until aromatic.

- In the pot, combine the washed lentils, water, vegetable broth, and bay leaf. To blend, stir.

- The soup should be brought to a boil, then simmer for 25 to 30 minutes, or until the lentils are soft, on low heat.

- Fresh spinach leaves should be added and cooked for a further two to three minutes, or until wilted.

- Add salt and pepper to taste and season the lentil soup.

- From the soup, remove the bay leaf.
- Pour some lemon juice over the heated lentil soup before serving. If you wish,

Quinoa and Roasted Vegetable Bowl

Ingredients:

Quinoa, one cup

2 cups of water or vegetable broth

1 sweet potato, chopped after peeling

1 diced red bell pepper

1 diced zucchini

1 thinly sliced, tiny red onion

Olive oil, two teaspoons

Oregano, dry, 1 teaspoon

of cumin, ground

pepper and salt as desired

For garnish, use fresh cilantro or parsley.

Method

- The oven should be preheated to 400°F (200°C).

- Put the quinoa through a cold water rinse.

- Quinoa and water or vegetable broth are combined in a pan. As soon as the mixture comes to a boil, turn down the heat, cover, and simmer for 15 to 20 minutes, or until the quinoa is tender and the liquid has been absorbed. With a fork, remove from the heat.

- On a baking sheet, distribute the diced sweet potato, zucchini, red bell pepper, and red onion.

- Sprinkle salt, pepper, ground cumin, dried oregano, and olive oil over the veggies. Even coat by tossing.

- The veggies should be roasted in a warm oven for 20 to 25 minutes, or until they are soft and just beginning to caramelize.

- Combine the cooked quinoa and roasted veggies in a serving dish.
- Garnish with fresh cilantro and parsley, if you wish.
- Warm up the dish of quinoa and vegetables before serving.
- Enjoy these healthy and tasty meals!

Chapter Four

Dinner Recipes

Salmon Baked with Roasted Veggies

Ingredients:

2 filets of salmon

Pepper and salt as desired

Olive oil, 1 tbsp

2 cups of chopped mixed veggies, including bell peppers, zucchini, and broccoli

One tablespoon of dried dill

Optional) Lemon wedges for serving

Method:

- Set the oven's temperature to 400°F (200°C).
- Add pepper and salt to the salmon fillets.
- In a skillet that is oven-safe, heat the olive oil over medium-high heat.

- The salmon fillets should be placed skin side down in the pan and seared for approximately 2 minutes, or until browned.
- Add the chopped mixed veggies to the pan after turning the salmon fillets over.
- On top of the salmon and veggies, scatter the dried dill.
- Once the salmon is cooked through and the veggies are soft, place the pan in the preheated oven and bake for 12 to 15 minutes.
- Take it out of the oven and give it some time to cool.
- With roasted veggies and, if preferred, a squeeze of lemon juice, serve the baked salmon.

Grilled Steak and Steamed Broccoli

Ingredients:

2 steaks, one inch thick, such as ribeye or sirloin

Pepper and salt as desired

Olive oil, 1 tbsp

200 grams of broccoli florets

Method:

- Set the grill's temperature to medium-high.
- Use pepper and salt to season the steaks.
- The steaks should be uniformly coated with the olive oil after being drizzled with it.
- For medium-rare doneness, place the steaks on the prepared grill and cook for approximately 4-5 minutes per side, or modify the cooking time to suit your preferences.

- Broccoli florets should be steamed until tender-crisp, approximately 5-7 minutes, in a steamer basket or saucepan with a little water while the steaks are cooking.
- After removing the steaks from the grill, give them some time to rest.
- Steamed broccoli should be served with the grilled steaks.

Brown rice with Stir-Fried Tofu

Ingredients:

1 block of cubed, firm, pressed tofu

2/4 cup soy sauce

One teaspoon of sesame oil

2 minced garlic cloves

1 teaspoon grated ginger

2 cups thinly sliced bell peppers, carrots, and other assorted stir-fry veggies

Vegetable oil, 1 tablespoon

2 cups of brown rice, cooked

Sesame seeds, and sliced green onions are optional garnishes.

Method

- Tofu cubes, soy sauce, and sesame oil should all be combined in a bowl. Give it around 15 minutes to marinate.
- In a large skillet or wok, warm the vegetable oil over medium-high heat.
- Stir-fry the grated ginger and minced garlic in the pan for approximately a minute, or until fragrant.
- Reserving the marinade, add the tofu that has been marinated to the pan. Stir-fry the tofu for 5 to 7 minutes, or until the exterior is slightly browned and crispy.
- When the veggies are tender-crisp, add the sliced stir-fry vegetables to the pan and stir-fry for an additional 3–4 minutes.

- Stirring to ensure a uniform coating, pour the reserved marinade over the tofu and veggies.

- Brown rice that has been cooked should be added to the pan and stir-fried for a few more minutes, or until everything is well heated.

- If preferred, top the hot brown rice with the stir-fried tofu and sprinkle with sesame seeds and thinly sliced green onions.

Spaghetti Squash with Turkey Meatballs

Ingredients:

Spaghetti squash, one

1 pound of turkey, ground

1/4 cup bread crumbs

Grated Parmesan cheese, 1/4 cup

Fresh parsley, chopped, one

Clove minced garlic, 1/4 cup

Oregano, dry, 1 teaspoon

One tablespoon dried basil

Pepper and salt as desired

2 cups of sauce marinara

Method:

- Set the oven's temperature to 400°F (200°C).

- Scoop out the seeds after cutting the spaghetti squash in half lengthwise.

- Squash halves should be placed cut-side down on a baking pan.

- When the squash is soft, bake it in the preheated oven for 40 to 45 minutes. Allow it to cool a little.

- Make the turkey meatballs while the squash bakes. Ground turkey, bread crumbs, grated Parmesan cheese, minced garlic, dried oregano, dried basil, salt, and pepper should all be combined in a bowl. Blend well.

- Create little meatballs out of the mixture.

- A big skillet with medium heat and one tablespoon of olive oil is heating.
- The turkey meatballs should be added to the pan and cooked for 8 to 10 minutes, or until browned and thoroughly cooked.
- The meatballs and marinara sauce should be combined in a pan, and the sauce should be heated through.
- Scrape the spaghetti squash strands that have been cooked onto a dish or plate using a fork.
- Serve the turkey meatballs and marinara sauce on top of the spaghetti squash.
- Enjoy making and eating these delectable dishes!

Chapter Five

Snacks and Appetizers

Crudité of Fresh Vegetables

Ingredients:

Banana sticks

Carrot sticks

Cut cucumbers

Bell pepper slices in a variety of hues

Plum tomatoes

Cauliflower florets

Broccoli florets

The dipping sauce of your choosing (such as ranch dressing or hummus)

Method

- The veggies should be washed and prepared by being chopped into sticks, slices, or florets.

- Place the vegetable crudité on separate serving plates or on a tray.
- Serve with a side of your preferred dipping sauce.
- Take pleasure in the crisp, fresh vegetables as an appetizer or nutritious snack.

Baked Sweet Potato Fries

Ingredients:

2 substantial sweet potatoes

Olive oil, two teaspoons

1 paprika teaspoon

One-half teaspoon of garlic powder

Pepper and salt as desired

Method

- A baking sheet should be lined with parchment paper, and the oven should be preheated to 425°F (220°C).

- The sweet potatoes should be peeled before being sliced into thin fries.
- Until they are well coated, mix the sweet potato fries in a bowl with olive oil, paprika, garlic powder, salt, and pepper.
- Place the fries on the baking sheet that has been prepared in a single layer.
- The fries should be crispy and golden brown after 20 to 25 minutes of baking in the preheated oven, turning halfway through.
- Before serving, take them out of the oven and allow them to cool somewhat.
- Enjoy the sweet potato fries cooked in place of conventional fries for a healthier option.

Fruit and Greek Yogurt Parfait

Ingredients

Greek yogurt, one cup

Mixed berries that are in season, including strawberries, blueberries, and raspberries

Honey or maple syrup for granola (optional)

Method

- Greek yogurt should be layered at the bottom of a glass or dish.
- To the yogurt, add a layer of mixed berries.
- Granola should be scattered on top of the fruit.
- The layers should be repeated until the glass or bowl is full.
- If you'd like, drizzle honey or maple syrup over top for more sweetness.
- Immediately serve the Greek yogurt and fruit parfait, or chill it until you're ready to eat.

Whole-Wheat Pita and Hummus

Ingredients:

Homemade or purchased hummus

Pita made of whole wheat, sliced into triangles
or wedges

Method:

- Put the hummus in a dish for serving.
- For dipping, cut the whole wheat pita
  bread into triangles or wedges.
- As a tasty and wholesome appetizer or
  snack, combine the whole wheat pita
  with hummus.
- Enjoy the savory whole wheat pita with
  creamy hummus for a pleasant meal.
- These dishes make excellent, healthy
  snacks or quick lunches. Enjoy!

Chapter Six

Desserts and Treats

Low-Sugar Berry Crumble:

Ingredients:

4 cups of mixed berries, including raspberries, blueberries, and strawberries

One teaspoon of lemon juice

1/4 cup almond meal

Oats, rolled, 1/4 cup

A quarter cup of chopped nuts, such as walnuts or almonds

2 teaspoons of coconut oil, melted

1 tablespoon maple syrup or honey (optional)

1 teaspoon of cinnamon powder

Method:

- An oven-safe baking dish should be lightly greased and heated to 350°F (175°C).

- Lemon juice and mixed berries should be combined in a dish. Toss the berries to cover them.

- Place the berries in the baking dish that has been buttered.

- Almond flour, rolled oats, chopped nuts, melted coconut oil, honey or maple syrup (if using), and ground cinnamon should all be well blended in a separate bowl.

- Over the berries, evenly distribute the crumble mixture.

- Bake for approximately 25 to 30 minutes in the preheated oven, or until the berries are bubbling and the crumble topping is golden.

- Before serving, take it out of the oven and allow it to cool somewhat.
- Warm sugar-free berry crumble may be served with a dollop of yogurt or a scoop of sugar-free ice cream, at your discretion.

Dark Chocolate Aavocado Mousse:

Ingredients:

Two mature avocados

Unsweetened cocoa powder, 1/4 cup

1/4 cup of melted dark chocolate chips

3 tablespoons of honey or maple syrup

One-half teaspoon of vanilla extract

A dash of salt

For a garnish, use chopped fresh berries or nuts.

Method:

- Cut the avocados in half, scoop out the meat, and discard the pits.

- The avocado flesh, cocoa powder, melted dark chocolate chips, maple syrup, honey, vanilla extract, and salt should all be combined in a blender or food processor.
- While processing, scrape down the edges as necessary to get a smooth, creamy texture.
- If necessary, taste and adjust the sweetness.
- Transfer the mousse made with dark chocolate and avocado to bowls or glasses for serving.
- Set it aside and chill in the refrigerator for at least an hour.
- Add fresh berries or chopped nuts as a garnish before serving, if preferred.
- Enjoy the delectable and healthy dessert choice of dark chocolate avocado mousse. It is rich and creamy.

Almond Flour Blueberry Muffins:

Ingredients:

Almond flour, two cups

1/4 cup coconut flour

1/4 cup maple syrup or honey

A quarter cup of melted coconut oil

Three big eggs

One tablespoon of baking powder

One-half teaspoon of vanilla extract

1 cup blueberries, either fresh or frozen

Method:

- Paper liners should be used to line a muffin pan while the oven is preheated to 350°F (175°C).
- Almond flour, coconut flour, baking powder, and a dash of salt should all be combined in a bowl.
- Melted coconut oil, eggs, honey or maple syrup, and vanilla extract should all be well blended in a different basin.

     Mclan O. Micheals, RDN.

- Mix all the dry ingredients with the addition of the liquid ones.
- Fold the blueberries in slowly.
- Spread the batter equally among the muffin tins that have been prepped, filling each one approximately 3/4 full.
- When the muffins are golden brown and a toothpick put in the middle of one comes out clean, bake them in the preheated oven for 20 to 25 minutes.
- After taking the muffins out of the oven, let them cool in the pan for a little while before moving them to a wire rack to finish cooling.
- Enjoy the blueberry muffins made with almond flour as a healthy, gluten-free breakfast or snack.

Baked Oatmeal Bars with Apple and Cinnamon:

Ingredients:

Rolled oats, 2 cups

Unsweetened applesauce, half a cup

1/4 cup maple syrup or honey

A quarter cup of melted coconut oil

Shredded and peeled apple, one big

1 cinnamon stick

A half-teaspoon of baking powder

1/4 teaspoon of salt

Topping: 1/4 cup chopped nuts (such as walnuts or almonds)

Method:

- An oven-safe baking dish should be lightly greased and heated to 350°F (175°C).

- Rolling oats, applesauce, honey or maple syrup, melted coconut oil, grated apple, cinnamon, baking soda, and salt should all be combined in a bowl. Stir well to mix.

- Spread out the oatmeal mixture equally in the oiled baking dish.
- For more crunch, if preferred, scatter the chopped nuts over top.
- When the oats are cooked through and the edges are golden brown, bake in the preheated oven for around 25 to 30 minutes.
- After taking it out of the oven, let it cool in the dish for a while before slicing it into bars or squares.
- The apple cinnamon baked oatmeal bars are a healthy and portable breakfast or snack. Serve warm.

Chapter Seven

Understanding Carbohydrate Counting

Certain foods naturally contain carbohydrates. For instance, the number of carbohydrates in grains, sweets, starches, legumes, and dairy varies. Learn about the three kinds of carbohydrates and the foods that contain each one.

The body's blood glucose, or blood sugar, level increases as a result of the digestion of carb-containing meals and beverages because the carbohydrates are converted into glucose, which powers our cells. Blood sugar levels increase after meals in people without diabetes, but the body's insulin response prevents levels from reaching too high.

If you have diabetes, the procedure doesn't operate as intended. Depending on your treatment plan and whether or not your body produces insulin, carb counting may or may not help you regulate your blood sugar levels.

     Mclan O. Micheals, RDN.

Type 1: If you have type 1 diabetes, your pancreas no longer produces insulin, so you must take background insulin in addition to doses of mealtime insulin to balance the carbohydrates in your diet.

Type 2: It's crucial to watch your carb consumption since individuals with type 2 diabetes may not create enough insulin and are resistant to it. Eating a constant quantity of carbohydrates at meals throughout the day rather than all at once will help prevent blood sugar increases. As opposed to people on insulin, individuals on oral medicines may use a simpler method of carb counting.

How are carbohydrates calculated?

At its most basic level, carb counting is calculating the amount of carbohydrates in a meal and comparing it to your insulin dosage.

If you use mealtime insulin, you must first calculate how many grams of carbohydrates you have consumed and then base your mealtime insulin dosage on that total. To determine how much insulin to take to control your blood sugar levels after eating, utilize a formula called an insulin-to-carb ratio. People with type 1 and some type 2 diabetes who are receiving intense insulin treatment through injections or pumps are advised to use this sophisticated method of carb counting.

While type 2 diabetics who don't use mealtime insulin may not need rigorous carb counting to maintain stable blood sugar levels, other individuals choose to. While some want to remain with the old method of counting carbohydrates, others prefer to use a simpler method based on "carbohydrate choices," where each "choice" has around 15 grams of carbohydrates. Others employ the Diabetes Plate Method, which recommends keeping whole grains, starchy vegetables, fruits, and dairy to a quarter of the plate, to consume an appropriate quantity of carb-containing items at each meal.

There are a few different approaches, and the ideal one for you will depend on your particular preferences and your demands in terms of your medications and way of life. You may get assistance determining what is best for you from a certified diabetes care and education specialist (CDCES) or a registered dietitian nutritionist (RDN/RD).

How much carbohydrate should I eat?

There is no magic number for how many carbohydrates should be consumed at each meal. Your body size and degree of exercise play a significant role in determining how much carbohydrate you require. Hunger and appetite also come into play.

You should first determine how many carbohydrates you currently consume at meals and snacks. You and your diabetes care team may learn a lot about how various meals affect your blood glucose by monitoring your food intake and your blood sugar before and approximately 2-3 hours after meals for a few days. This can help you identify the appropriate quantity of carbohydrates for you.

How much carbohydrate is in my food?

Reading food labels will reveal how many carbohydrates are present in foods. There are applications and other tools available to help you determine whether a product, such as a whole fruit or vegetable, lacks a food label. The good news is that you'll recall the carbohydrate amounts of the meals you often consume better the longer you practice carb counting.

When calculating carbs, you should focus on the following two things on the nutrition information label:

All of the information on the label pertains to this exact quantity of food, which is referred to as the serving size. You must take into consideration the extra nutrients if you consume more. For instance, if you consume two or three servings of anything, you will need to multiply by two or three the grams of carbohydrates (as well as all other nutrients) listed on the label. This sums up all carbohydrates, including fiber, starch, and sugar. That's correct, the overall amount of carbohydrates already includes the grams of added sugars, so you don't need to worry about putting them on. To give you a better idea of what's in the meal you're consuming, there are additional bullets listed underneath the total number of carbohydrates. And although while added sugars aren't a concern when it comes to counting carbohydrates, you should still make an effort to limit their presence in your diet.

Chapter Eight

Conclusion

Being a newly diagnosed man with diabetes may provide its fair share of difficulties and adjustments. You must keep in mind that you are not traveling this route alone. Diabetes management with a healthy diet may become automatic with the correct information, resources, and support, empowering you to take charge of your health and lead a satisfying lifestyle.

We have created a variety of tasty and nourishing dishes. This cookbook provides a broad range of delectable selections to suit your preferences, from robust breakfast options to filling lunches and dinners, and even decadent but diabetes-friendly desserts.

Along with the recipes, we also included helpful advice on reading labels, portion management, understanding carbs, and meal planning. You may make wise decisions, efficiently control your blood sugar levels, and maintain a healthy weight by adopting these tactics into your everyday routine.

Keep in mind that this book is not intended to be a one-size-fits-all answer. Each person's experience with diabetes is distinct, so it's important to collaborate closely with your medical team to create a tailored strategy that meets your particular requirements. Regular checkups, blood sugar testing, and medication alterations as required are essential components of managing your diabetes.

Never forget that controlling diabetes is a lifetime commitment. Although it may have its ups and downs, you may have a happy, healthy life if you are determined, knowledgeable, and optimistic. If you embrace the power of proper diet, exercise, and self-care, you'll discover that managing your diabetes successfully is not only feasible but also empowering.

Take advantage of the delectable dishes, accept the insightful advice, and take control of your diabetes care. You have the ability to prosper, live well, and take advantage of everything that life has to offer.

I wish you good health, joy, and success as you work to live a balanced and rewarding life while having diabetes!

21 Days Meal Plan

Day 1:

Breakfast: A nutritious meal Bowl
Lunch: Grilled chicken salad
Dinner: Roasted vegetables and baked salmon.

Day 2:

Breakfast: Eggs with vegetables
Lunch: Turkey and Veggie Wrap
Dinner: Grilled steak and steamed broccoli.

Day 3

Breakfast: Whole grain pancakes
Lunch: Lentil soup with spinach
Dinner: Brown rice with Stir-Fried Tofu

Day 4

Breakfast: Poached eggs and avocado toast
Lunch: Quinoa and Roasted Vegetable Bowl
Dinner: Spaghetti Squash and Turkey Meatballs

Day 5

Breakfast: Fresh vegetable crudités
Lunch: Baked sweet potato fries
Dinner: Greek yogurt and fruit parfait

Day 6
Breakfast: Grilled chicken salad for breakfast
Lunch: Vegetable omelet for lunch
Dinner: Roasted vegetables and baked salmon.

Day 7
Breakfast: A nutritious meal Bowl
Lunch: Turkey and Veggie Wrap
Dinner: Grilled Steak and Steamed Broccoli

Day 8
Breakfast: Whole grain pancakes
Lunch: Lentil soup with spinach
Dinner: Brown rice with Stir-Fried Tofu

Day 9
Breakfast: Poached eggs and avocado toast
Lunch: Quinoa and Roasted Vegetable Bowl
Dinner: Spaghetti Squash and Turkey Meatballs

Day 10
Breakfast: Fresh vegetable crudités
Lunch: Baked sweet potato fries for lunch
Dinner: Greek yogurt and fruit parfait

Day 11
Breakfast: Grilled chicken salad

Lunch: Vegetable omelet for lunch
Dinner: Roasted vegetables and baked salmon.

Day 12
Breakfast: A nutritious meal Bowl
Lunch: Turkey and Veggie Wrap
Dinner: Grilled Steak and Steamed Broccoli

Day 13
Breakfast: Whole grain pancakes
Lunch: Lentil soup with spinach
Dinner: Brown rice with Stir-Fried Tofu

Day 14
Breakfast: Poached eggs and avocado toast
Lunch: Quinoa and Roasted Vegetable Bowl
Dinner: Spaghetti Squash and Turkey Meatballs

Day 15
Breakfast: Fresh vegetable crudités
Lunch: Baked sweet potato fries
Dinner: Greek yogurt and fruit parfait

Day 16
Breakfast: Grilled chicken salad
Lunch: Vegetable omelet
Dinner: Roasted vegetables and baked salmon.

Day 17
Breakfast: A nutritious meal Bowl
Lunch: Turkey and Veggie Wrap
Dinner: Grilled Steak and Steamed Broccoli

Day 18
Breakfast: Whole grain pancakes
Lunch: Lentil soup with spinach
Dinner: Brown rice with Stir-Fried Tofu

Day 19
Breakfast: Poached eggs and avocado toast
Lunch: Quinoa and Roasted Vegetable Bowl
Dinner: Spaghetti Squash and Turkey Meatballs

Day 20
Breakfast: Fresh vegetable crudités
Lunch: Baked sweet potato fries
Dinner: Greek yogurt and fruit parfait

Day 21:
Breakfast: Grilled chicken salad
Lunch: Vegetable omelet for lunch
Dinner: Roasted vegetables and baked salmon.

You are welcome to modify this menu to suit your tastes and dietary requirements.